Hailing from Denver, Colorado Kendall is a YouTube [s] crime, mystery and conspiracy videos. She also cohosts husband, Josh, called the Mile Higher Podcast. Across a [platf]orms she has over 1 milllion followers and counting. She is an aavocate for missing persons and uses her platform to raise money and awareness for Thorn which is a non-profit international anti-human trafficking organization founded by Ashton Kutcher and Demi Moore.

Kendall aims to inspire, educate, and promote critical thinking while making complicated topics more interesting and easy to grasp. She focuses on true crime, unsolved mysteries, astrology, conspiracies, space exploration, suspenseful stories, ancient history, personal topics, and promotion of better care for the planet and mental health. She is loved by her audience for being very down to earth, relatable, and genuine.

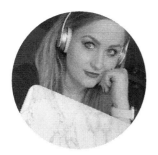

Kendall Rae

P.S. Thank you so much for purchasing my coloring book. If you enjoyed this book please leave us a review on Amazon.

Happy Coloring!

Follow on social networks:
youtube.com/KendallsPlace
youtube.com/milehigherpodcast
twitter.com/kendallraeonyt
twitter.com/milehigherpod
instagram.com/milehigherpodcast
milehigherpodcast.com
milehighermerch.com
milehighermedia.com

COLOR TEST PAGE

Use this test page to try out different colors and mediums.

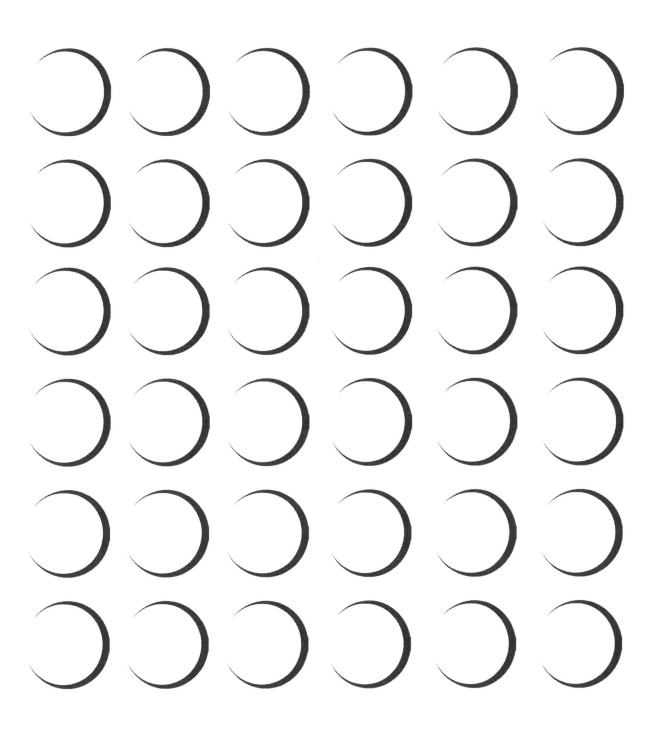

"

Everything around you that you call life was made up by people that were no smarter than you, and you can **change it**, you can **influence it**, you can build your own things that other people can use. - **Steve Jobs**

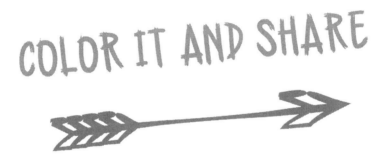

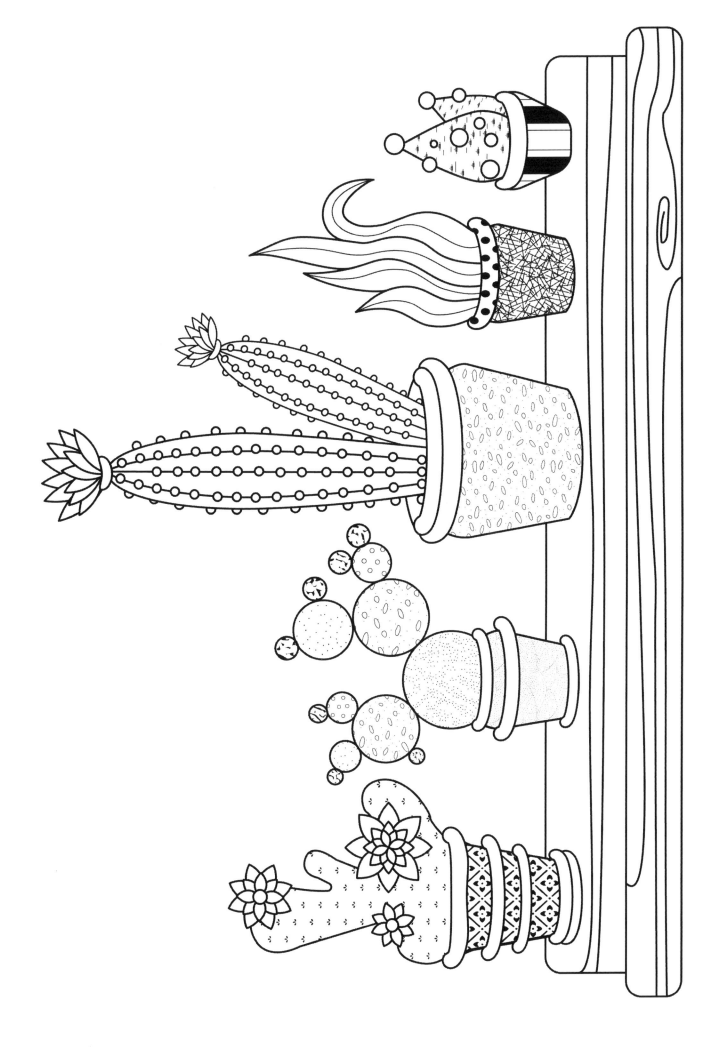

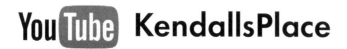

This page is left BLANK intentionally to avoid any bleed-through on the paper.

Thank you so much for purchasing my coloring book.
If you enjoyed this book please leave us a review on Amazon.

We want to see your drawings. Send us your colored version and tag us!

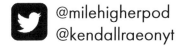 @milehigherpod
@kendallraeonyt

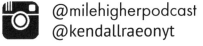 @milehigherpodcast
@kendallraeonyt

"
Our entire biological system, the brain and the earth itself work on the same frequencies.
-**Nikola Tesla**

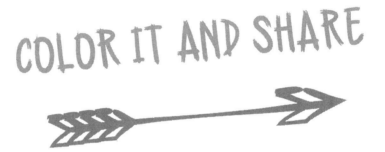

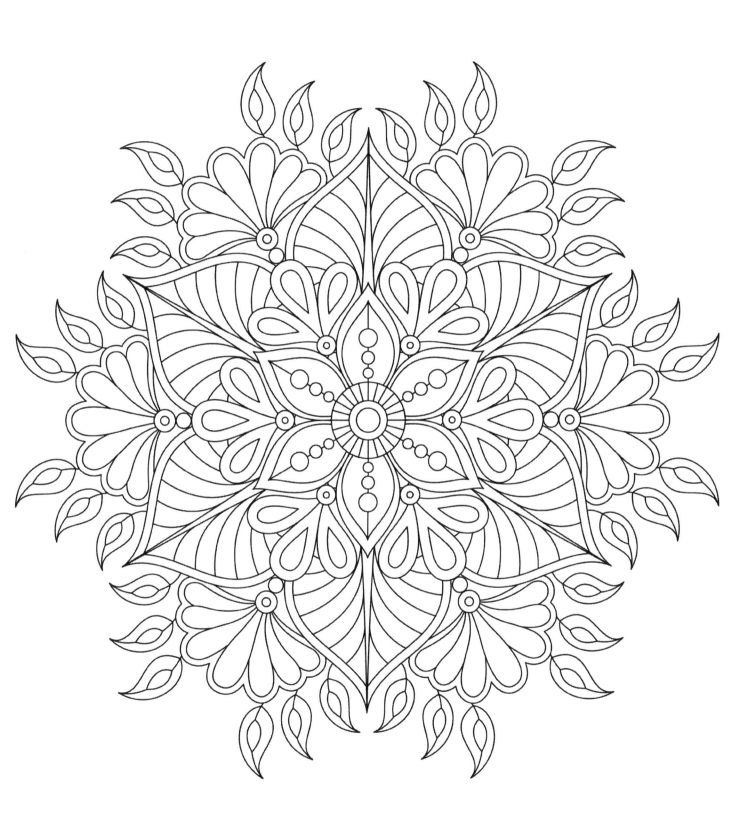

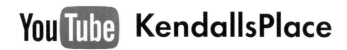

This page is left BLANK intentionally to avoid any bleed-through on the paper.

Thank you so much for purchasing my coloring book.
If you enjoyed this book please leave us a review on Amazon.

We want to see your drawings. Send us your colored version and tag us!

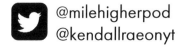 @milehigherpod
@kendallraeonyt

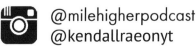 @milehigherpodcast
@kendallraeonyt

You were born an **orignal**. Don't die a copy.
- **John Mason**

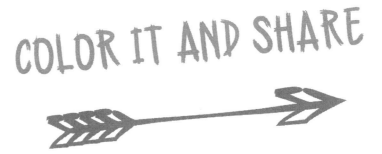

Want to get more free printable sheets? Get it here:
www.kendallr.com

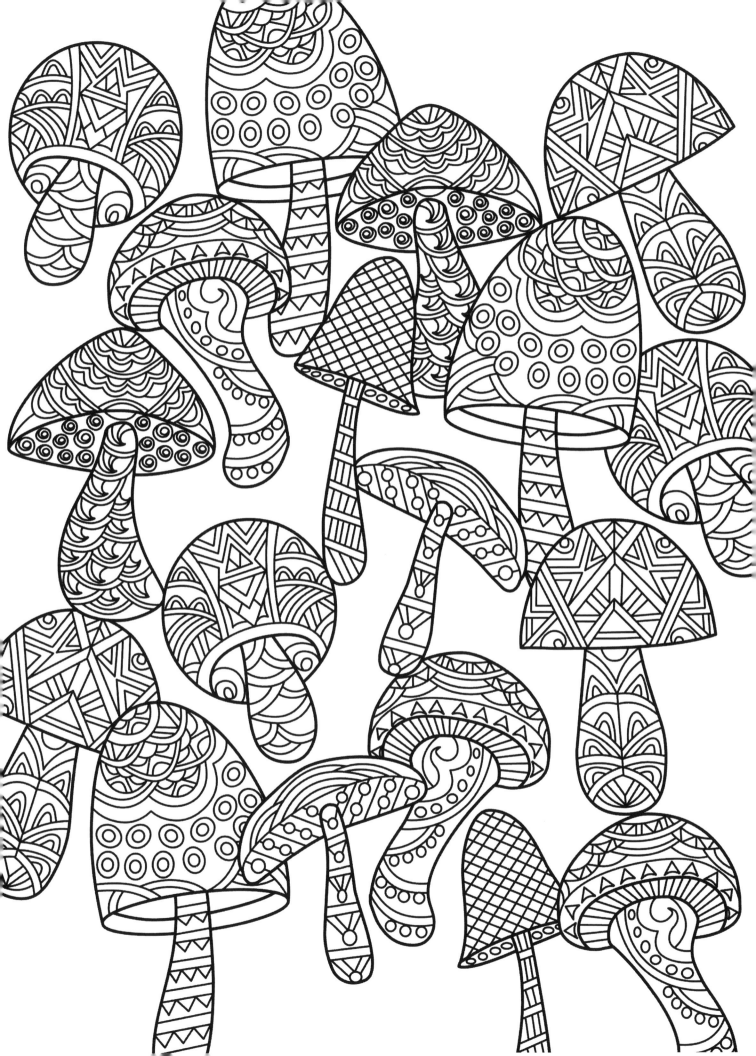

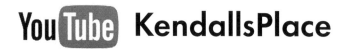

This page is left BLANK intentionally to avoid any bleed-through on the paper.

Thank you so much for purchasing my coloring book.
If you enjoyed this book please leave us a review on Amazon.

To **be creative** is to let little pieces of your heart go & place them into each project you make. - **Pat Bravo**

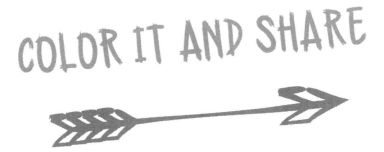

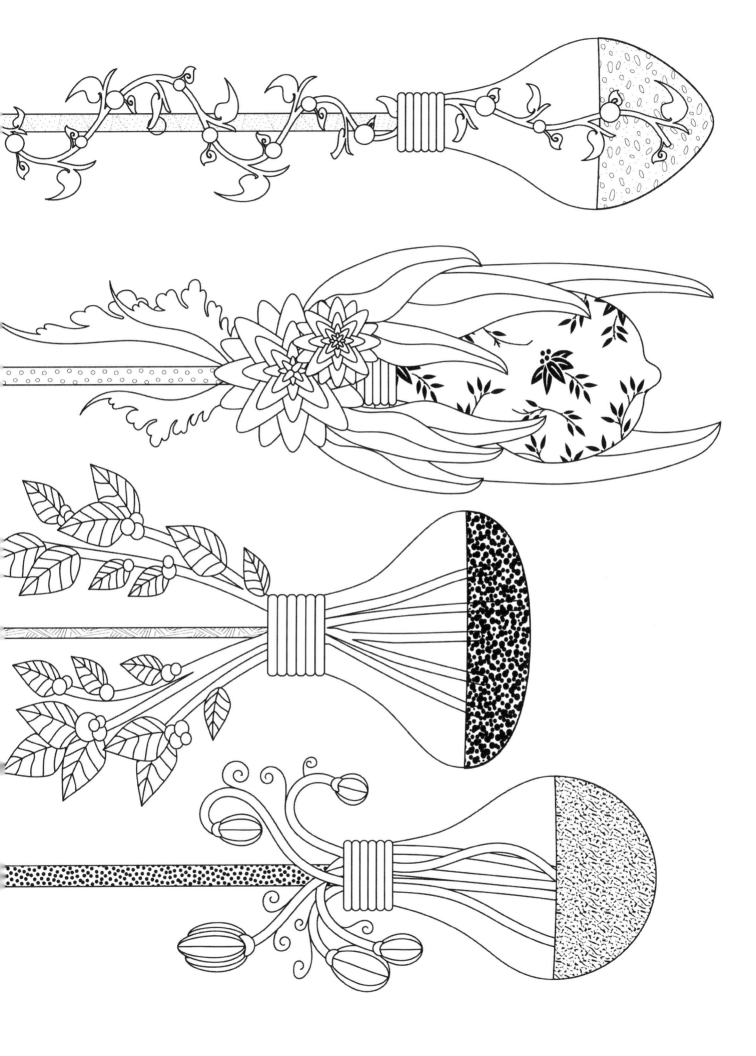

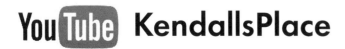

This page is left BLANK intentionally to avoid any bleed-through on the paper.

Thank you so much for purchasing my coloring book.
If you enjoyed this book please leave us a review on Amazon.

We want to see your drawings. Send us your colored version and tag us!

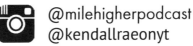

@milehigherpod   @milehigherpodcast
@kendallraeonyt   @kendallraeonyt

"

With freedom, books, flowers, and the moon, who could not be happy?

- **Oscar Wilde**

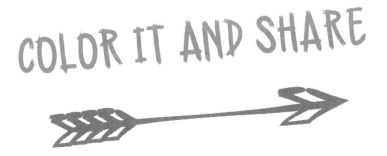

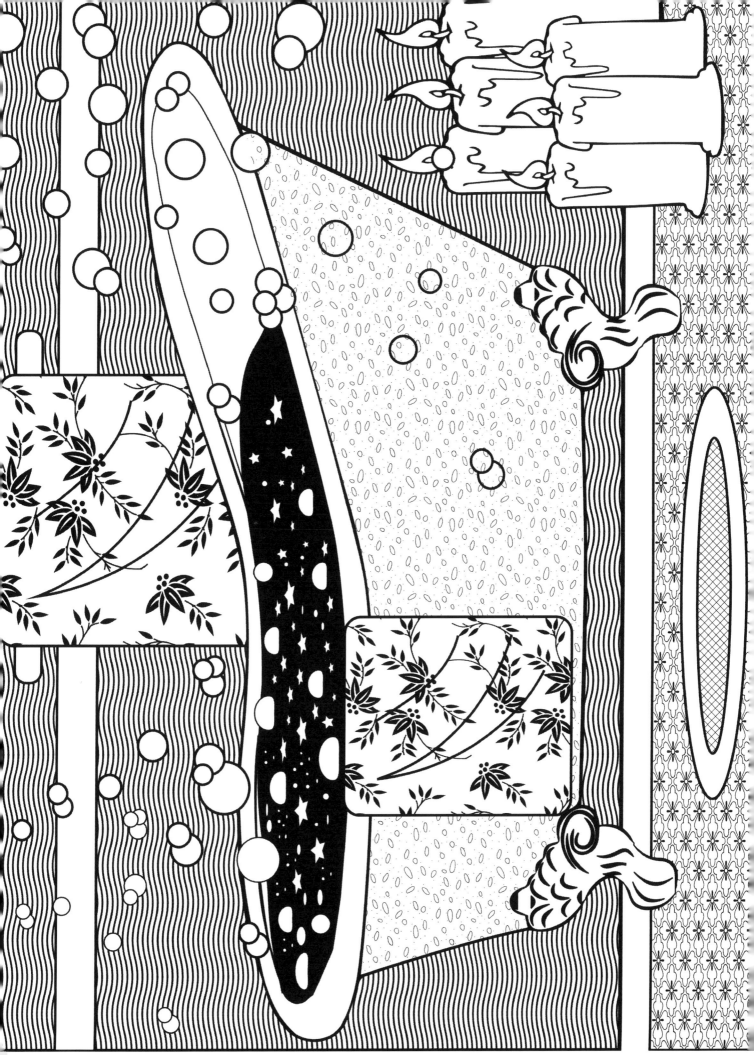

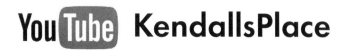

This page is left BLANK intentionally to avoid any bleed-through on the paper.

Thank you so much for purchasing my coloring book.
If you enjoyed this book please leave us a review on Amazon.

We want to see your drawings. Send us your colored version and tag us!

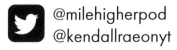 @milehigherpod
@kendallraeonyt

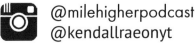 @milehigherpodcast
@kendallraeonyt

"Everything you want is on the other side of fear. - **Jack Canfield**

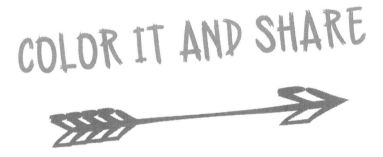

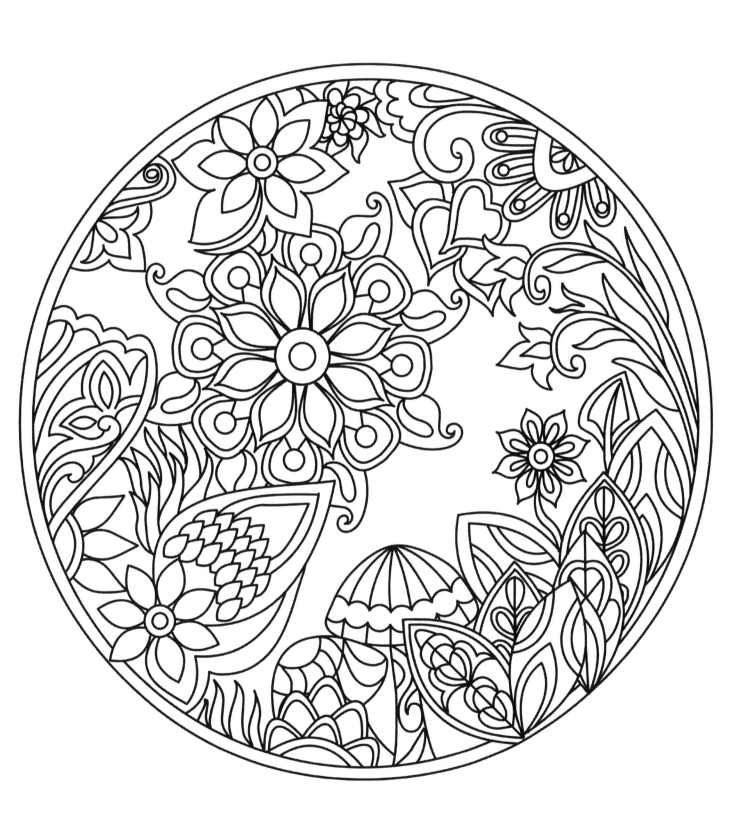

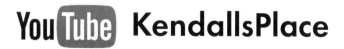

This page is left BLANK intentionally to avoid any bleed-through on the paper.

Thank you so much for purchasing my coloring book.
If you enjoyed this book please leave us a review on Amazon.

We want to see your drawings. Send us your colored version and tag us!

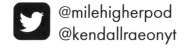 @milehigherpod
@kendallraeonyt

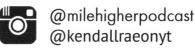 @milehigherpodcast
@kendallraeonyt

"If you are always trying to be normal, you will never know how **amazing** you can be. - **Maya Angelou**

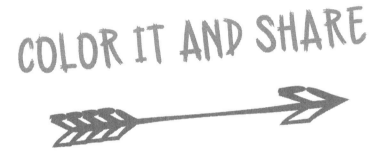

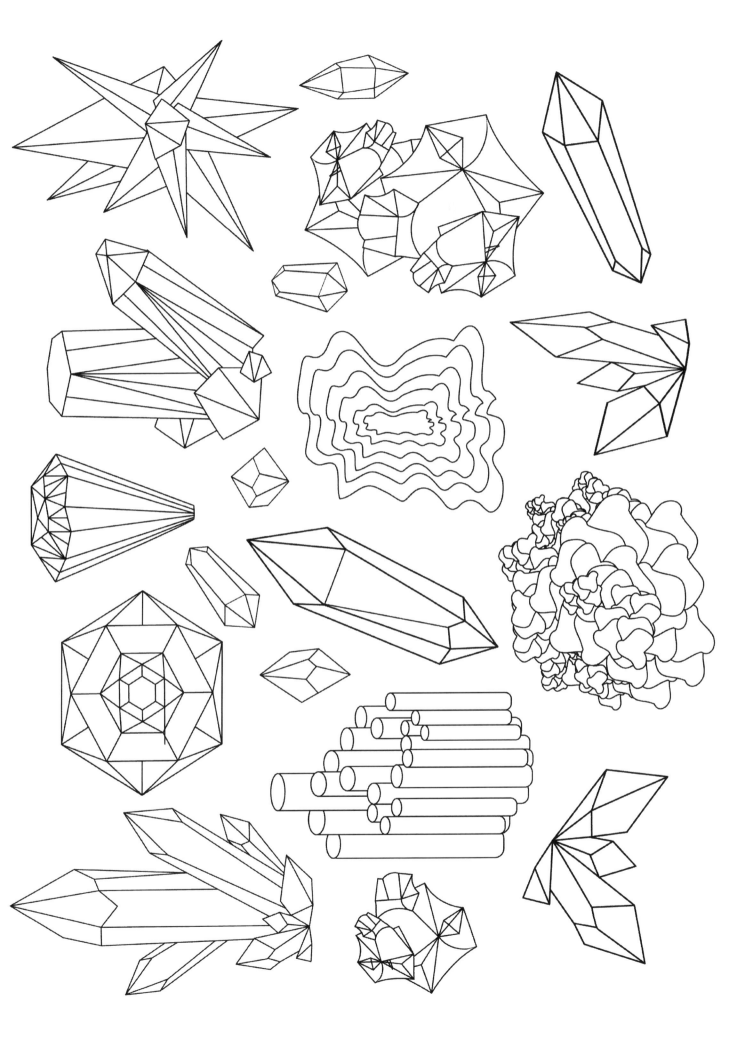

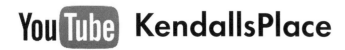

This page is left BLANK intentionally to avoid any bleed-through on the paper.

Thank you so much for purchasing my coloring book.
If you enjoyed this book please leave us a review on Amazon.

We want to see your drawings. Send us your colored version and tag us!

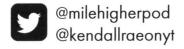 @milehigherpod
@kendallraeonyt

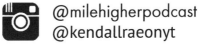 @milehigherpodcast
@kendallraeonyt

"Doubt kills more **dreams** than failure ever will.
-**Karim Seddiki**

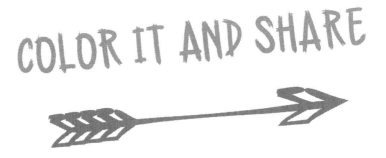

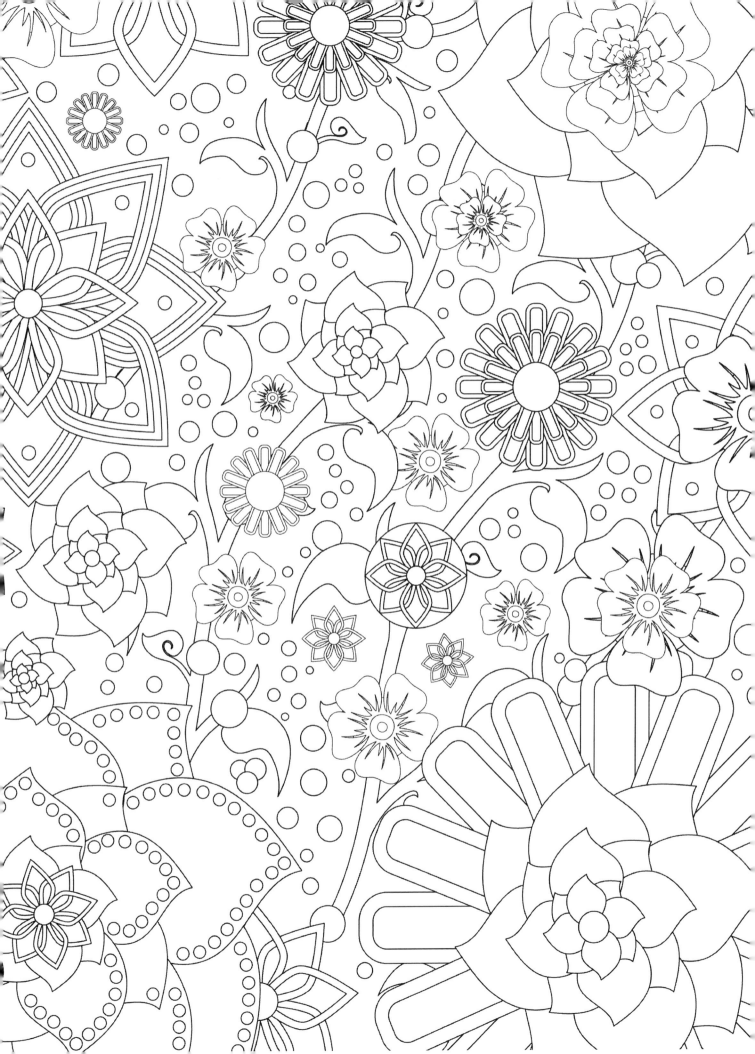

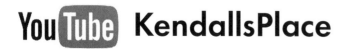

This page is left BLANK intentionally to avoid any bleed-through on the paper.

Thank you so much for purchasing my coloring book.
If you enjoyed this book please leave us a review on Amazon.

We want to see your drawings. Send us your colored version and tag us!

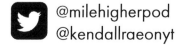 @milehigherpod
@kendallraeonyt

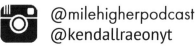 @milehigherpodcast
@kendallraeonyt

"

The **soul**, **creativity** or **love** put into something; the essence of yourself that is put into your work. - **Meraki (n.)**

COLOR IT AND SHARE

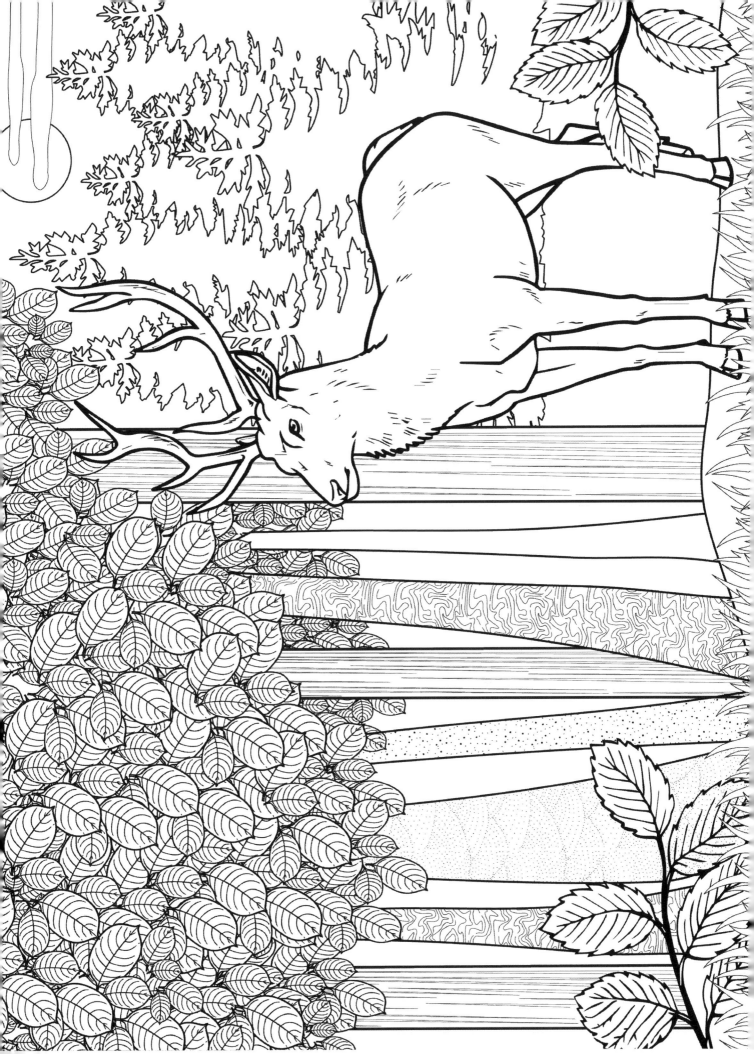

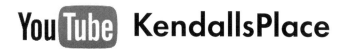

This page is left BLANK intentionally to avoid any bleed-through on the paper.

Thank you so much for purchasing my coloring book.
If you enjoyed this book please leave us a review on Amazon.

We want to see your drawings. Send us your colored version and tag us!

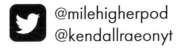 @milehigherpod
@kendallraeonyt

 @milehigherpodcast
@kendallraeonyt

" If you're not doing what you **love**, you're wasting your time. - **Billy Joel**

COLOR IT AND SHARE

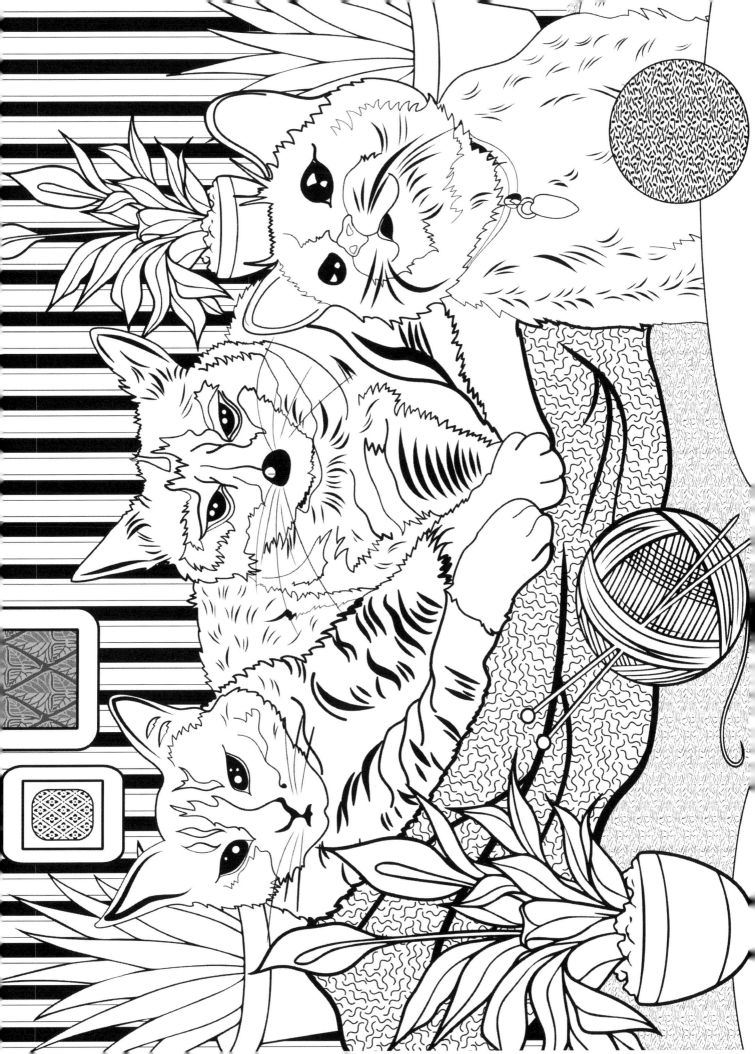

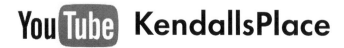

This page is left BLANK intentionally to avoid any bleed-through on the paper.

Thank you so much for purchasing my coloring book.
If you enjoyed this book please leave us a review on Amazon.

We want to see your drawings. Send us your colored version and tag us!

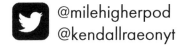 @milehigherpod
@kendallraeonyt

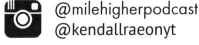 @milehigherpodcast
@kendallraeonyt

"**Cloud walker**"; one who lives in the clouds of their own imagination or dreams or one who does not obey the conventions of society, literature, or art. - **Nefelibata (n.) Lit.**

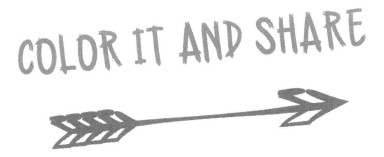

Want to get more free printable sheets? Get it here:
www.kendallr.com

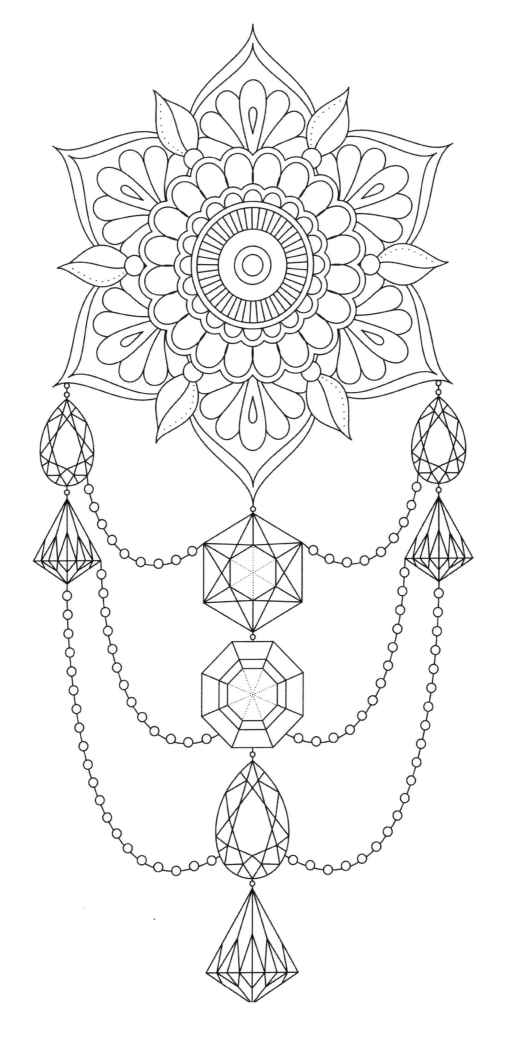

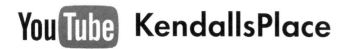

This page is left BLANK intentionally to avoid any bleed-through on the paper.

Thank you so much for purchasing my coloring book.
If you enjoyed this book please leave us a review on Amazon.

We want to see your drawings. Send us your colored version and tag us!

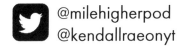 @milehigherpod
@kendallraeonyt

 @milehigherpodcast
@kendallraeonyt

"

Calm mind brings inner strength and self-confidence, so that's very important for good health. - **Dalai Lama**

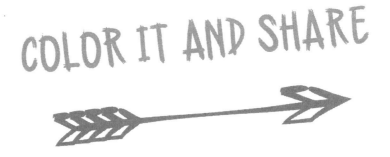

This page is left BLANK intentionally to avoid any bleed-through on the paper.

Thank you so much for purchasing my coloring book.
If you enjoyed this book please leave us a review on Amazon.

We want to see your drawings. Send us your colored version and tag us!

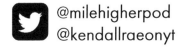 @milehigherpod
@kendallraeonyt

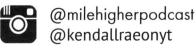 @milehigherpodcast
@kendallraeonyt

Quality is not an act, it is a **habit** - **Aristotle**

COLOR IT AND SHARE

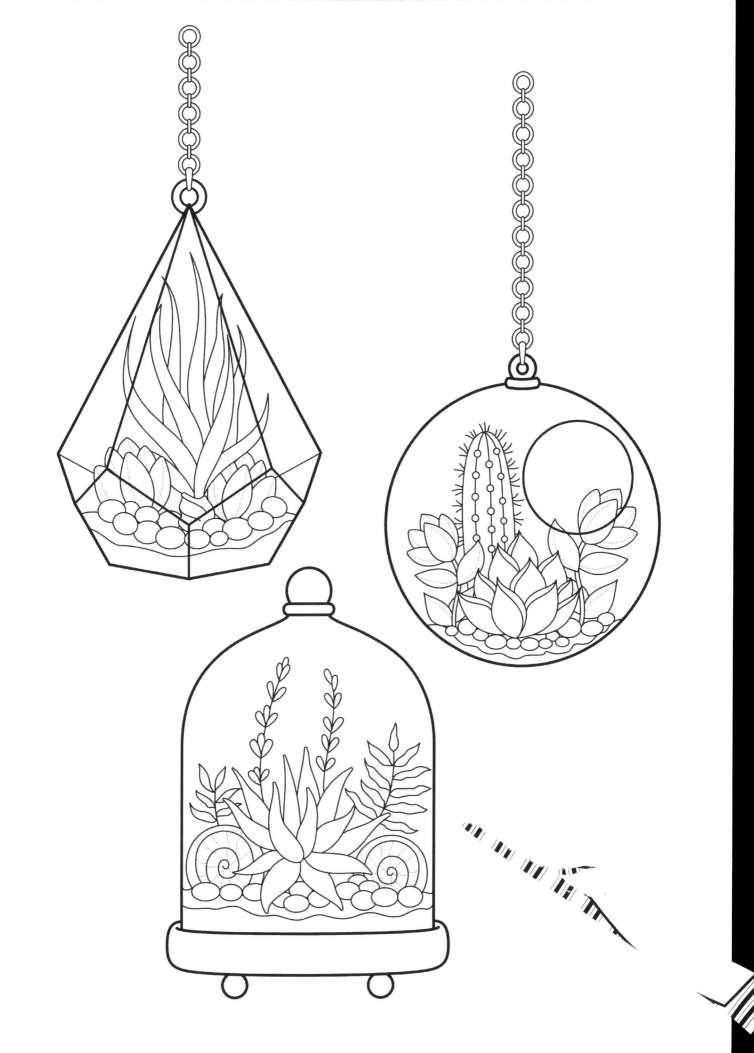

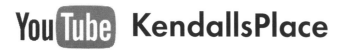

This page is left BLANK intentionally to avoid any bleed-through on the paper.

Thank you so much for purchasing my coloring book.
If you enjoyed this book please leave us a review on Amazon.

We want to see your drawings. Send us your colored version and tag us!

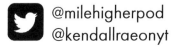 @milehigherpod
@kendallraeonyt

 @milehigherpodcast
@kendallraeonyt

"Well **done** is better than well said - **Benjamin Franklin**

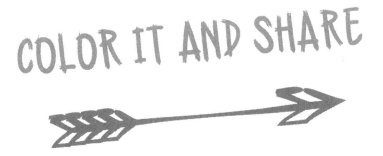

Want to get more free printable sheets? Get it here:
www.kendallr.com

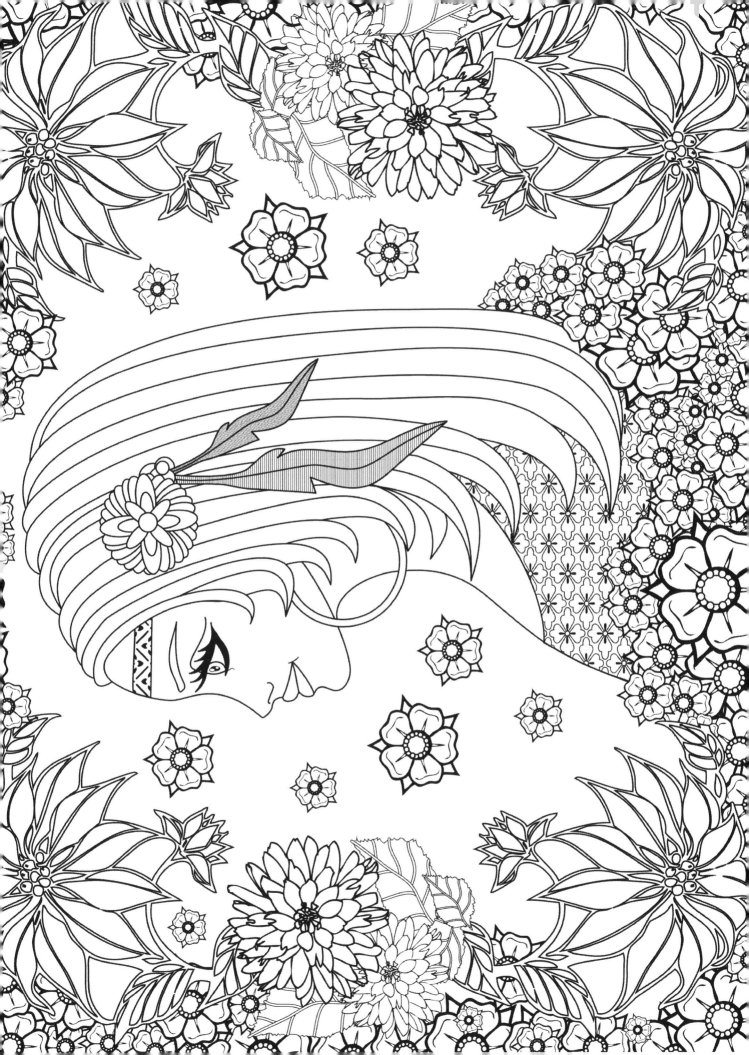

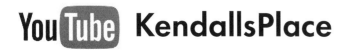

This page is left BLANK intentionally to avoid any bleed-through on the paper.

Thank you so much for purchasing my coloring book.
If you enjoyed this book please leave us a review on Amazon.

We want to see your drawings. Send us your colored version and tag us!

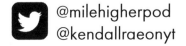 @milehigherpod
@kendallraeonyt

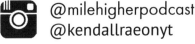 @milehigherpodcast
@kendallraeonyt

You don't have to be great to start, but you have to **start** to be great - **Zig Ziglar**

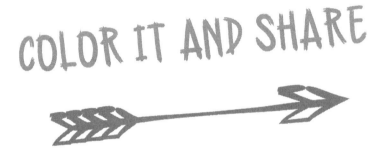

Want to get more free printable sheets? Get it here:
www.kendallr.com

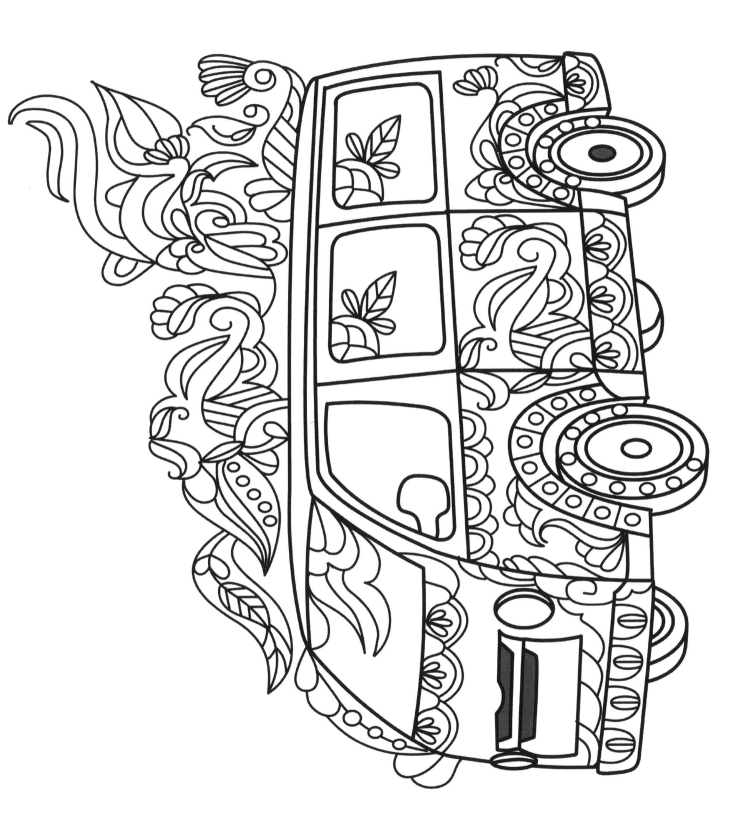

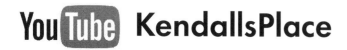

This page is left BLANK intentionally to avoid any bleed-through on the paper.

Thank you so much for purchasing my coloring book.
If you enjoyed this book please leave us a review on Amazon.

We want to see your drawings. Send us your colored version and tag us!

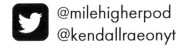 @milehigherpod
@kendallraeonyt

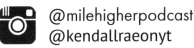 @milehigherpodcast
@kendallraeonyt

Success is walking from failure to failure with no loss of enthusiasm. - **Winston Churchill**

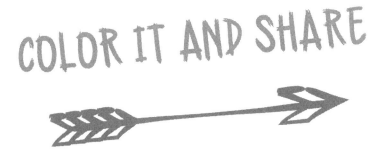

Want to get more free printable sheets? Get it here:
www.kendallr.com

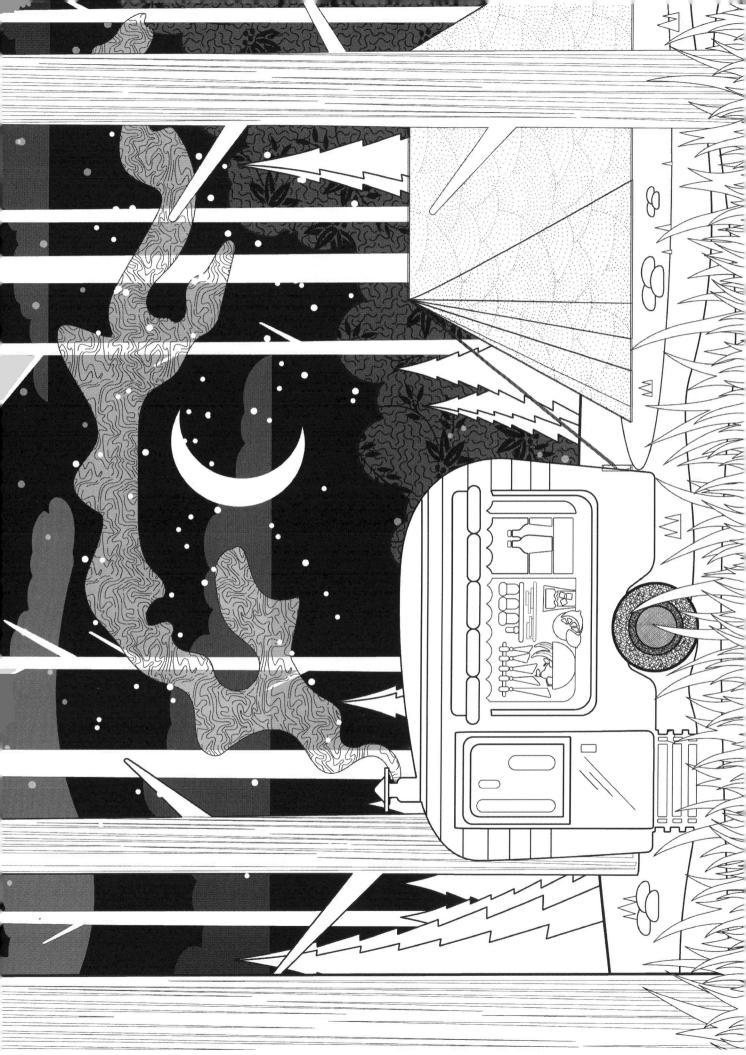

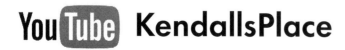

This page is left BLANK intentionally to avoid any bleed-through on the paper.

Thank you so much for purchasing my coloring book.
If you enjoyed this book please leave us a review on Amazon.

We want to see your drawings. Send us your colored version and tag us!

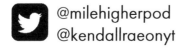 @milehigherpod
@kendallraeonyt

 @milehigherpodcast
@kendallraeonyt

The secret of getting ahead is **getting started**. - **Mark Twain**

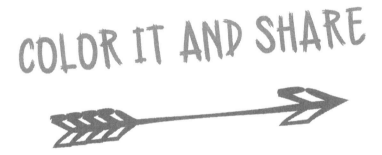

Want to get more free printable sheets? Get it here:
www.kendallr.com

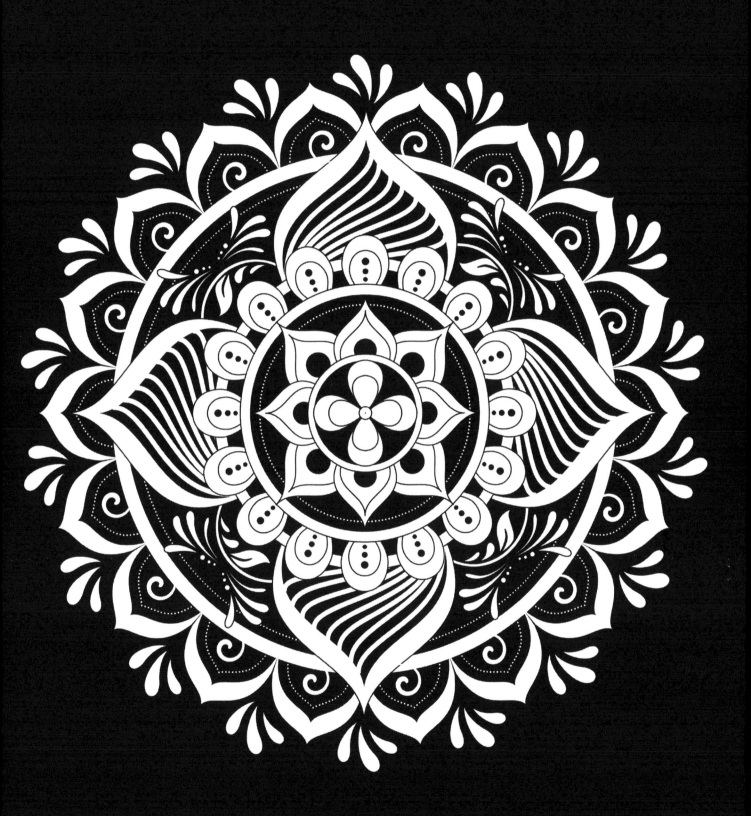

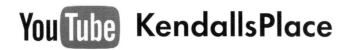

This page is left BLANK intentionally to avoid any bleed-through on the paper.

Thank you so much for purchasing my coloring book.
If you enjoyed this book please leave us a review on Amazon.

We want to see your drawings. Send us your colored version and tag us!

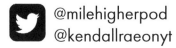 @milehigherpod
@kendallraeonyt

 @milehigherpodcast
@kendallraeonyt

> "Don't watch the clock; do what it does. **Keep going.** - Sam Levenson

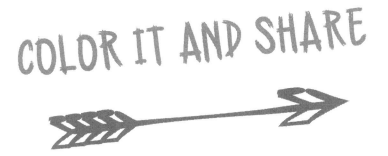

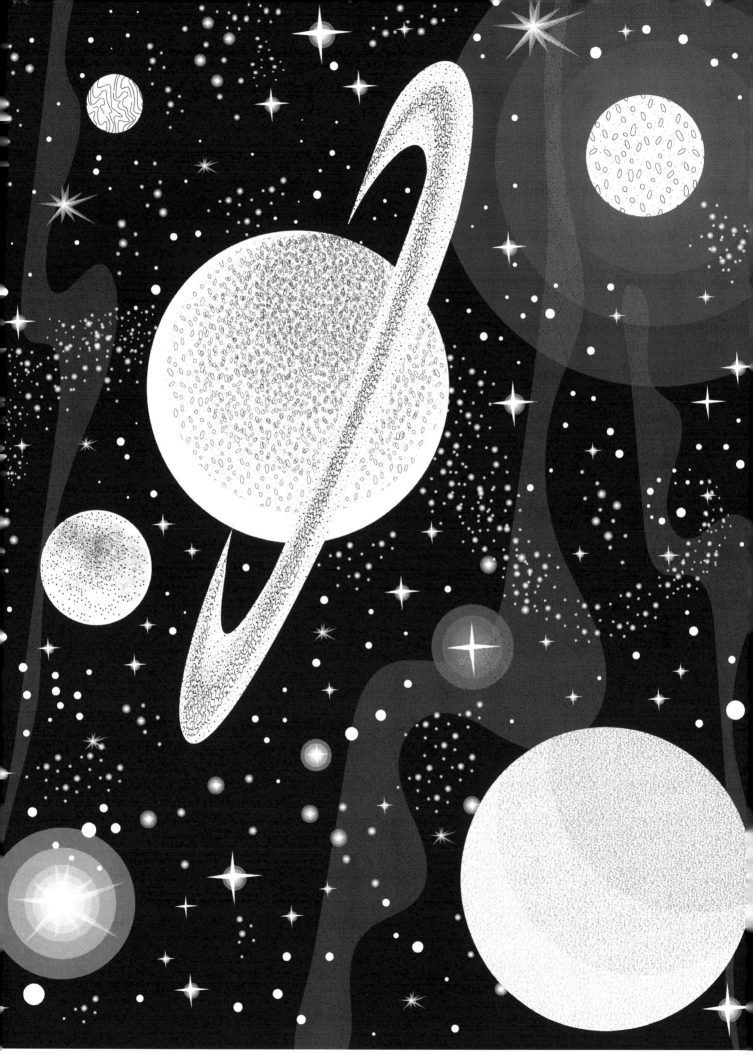

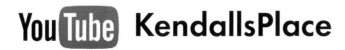

This page is left BLANK intentionally to avoid any bleed-through on the paper.

Thank you so much for purchasing my coloring book.
If you enjoyed this book please leave us a review on Amazon.

We want to see your drawings. Send us your colored version and tag us!

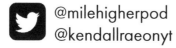 @milehigherpod
@kendallraeonyt

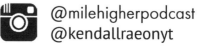 @milehigherpodcast
@kendallraeonyt

"

Too many of us are not living our **dreams** because we are living our fears. - **Les Brown**

COLOR IT AND SHARE

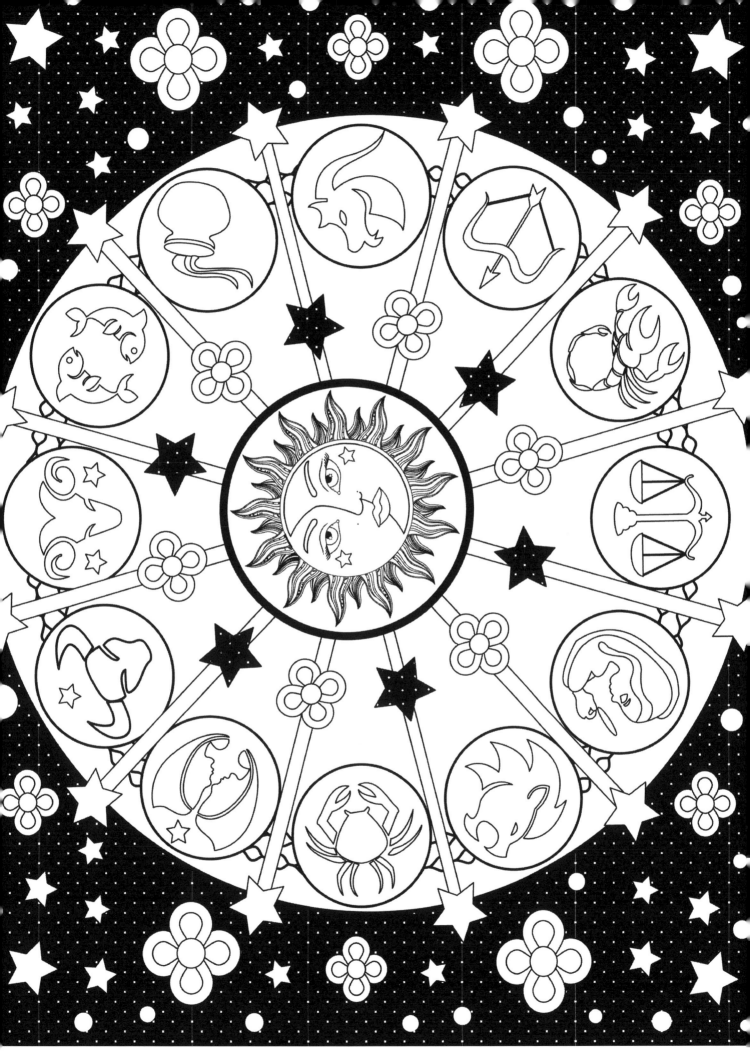

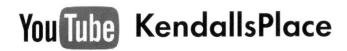

This page is left BLANK intentionally to avoid any bleed-through on the paper.

Thank you so much for purchasing my coloring book.
If you enjoyed this book please leave us a review on Amazon.

We want to see your drawings. Send us your colored version and tag us!

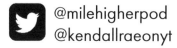 @milehigherpod
@kendallraeonyt

 @milehigherpodcast
@kendallraeonyt

" Either I will find a way or I **will make** one -
Philip Sidney

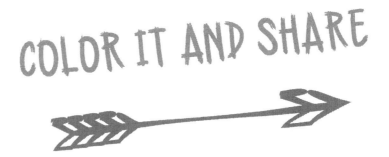

Want to get more free printable sheets? Get it here:
www.kendallr.com

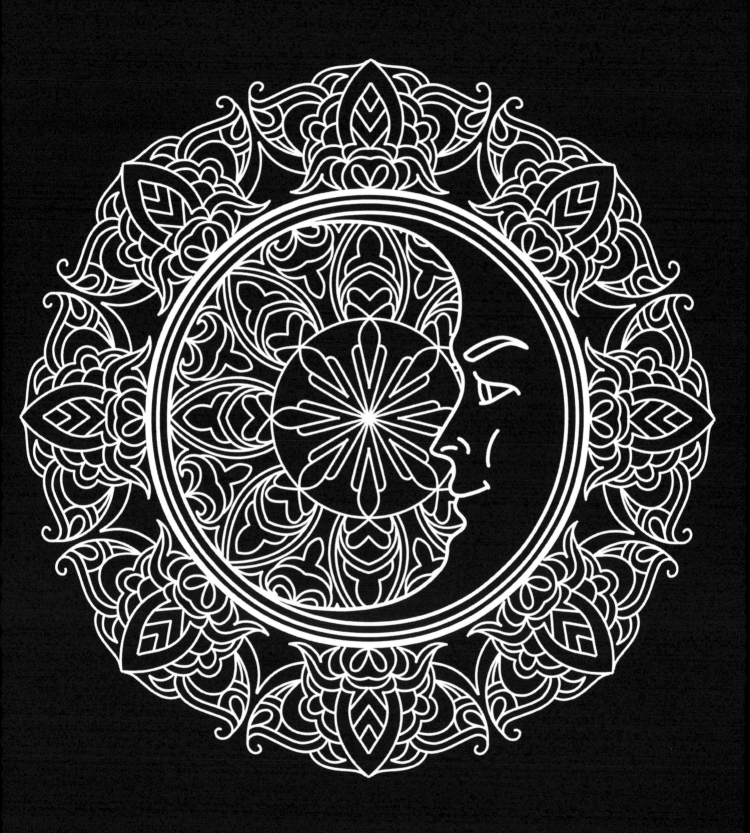

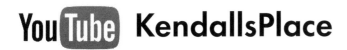

This page is left BLANK intentionally to avoid any bleed-through on the paper.

Thank you so much for purchasing my coloring book.
If you enjoyed this book please leave us a review on Amazon.

We want to see your drawings. Send us your colored version and tag us!

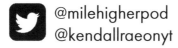 @milehigherpod
@kendallraeonyt

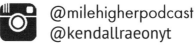 @milehigherpodcast
@kendallraeonyt

"

After a storm comes a **calm** - **Matthew Henry**

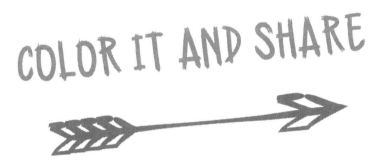

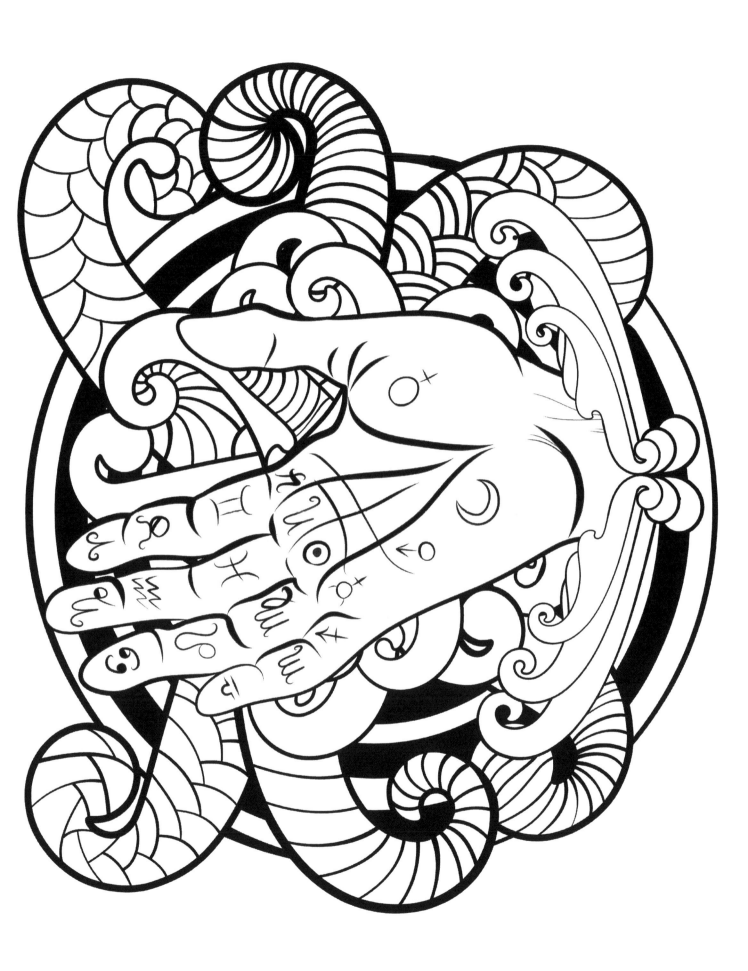

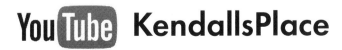

This page is left BLANK intentionally to avoid any bleed-through on the paper.

Thank you so much for purchasing my coloring book.
If you enjoyed this book please leave us a review on Amazon.

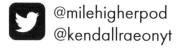
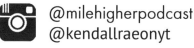

"

Hitch your wagon to a **star** - **Ralph Waldo Emerson**

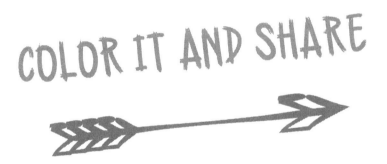

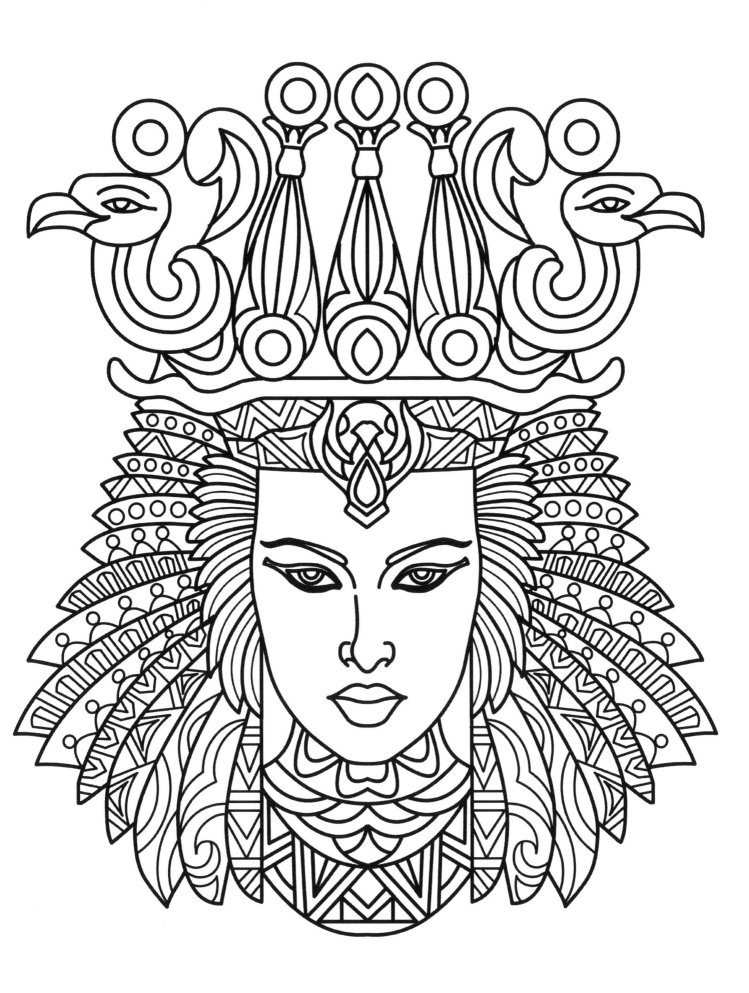

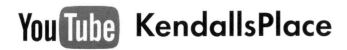

This page is left BLANK intentionally to avoid any bleed-through on the paper.

Thank you so much for purchasing my coloring book.
If you enjoyed this book please leave us a review on Amazon.

We want to see your drawings. Send us your colored version and tag us!

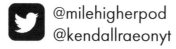 @milehigherpod
@kendallraeonyt

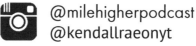 @milehigherpodcast
@kendallraeonyt

Either **move** or be moved - **Ezra Pound**

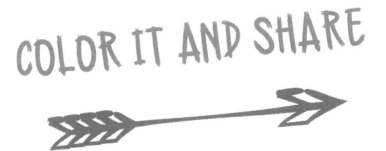

Want to get more free printable sheets? Get it here:
www.kendallr.com

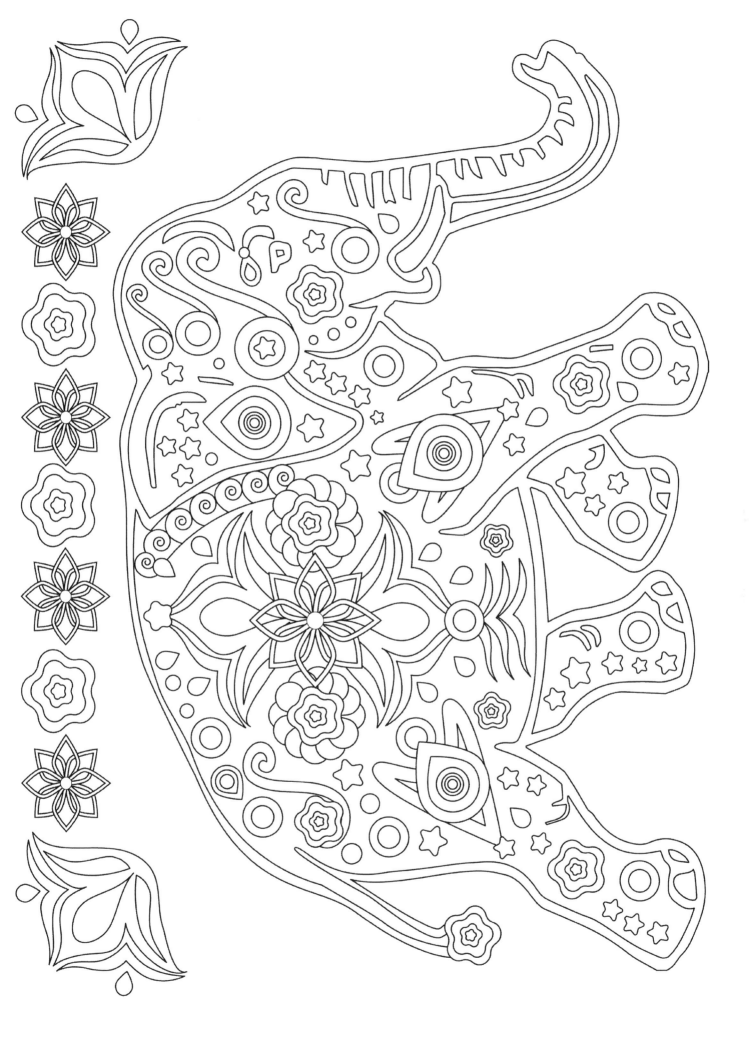

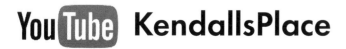

This page is left BLANK intentionally to avoid any bleed-through on the paper.

Thank you so much for purchasing my coloring book.
If you enjoyed this book please leave us a review on Amazon.

We want to see your drawings. Send us your colored version and tag us!

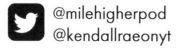 @milehigherpod
@kendallraeonyt

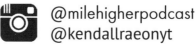 @milehigherpodcast
@kendallraeonyt

" "

Do whatever you do **intensely**. - **Robert Henri**

COLOR IT AND SHARE

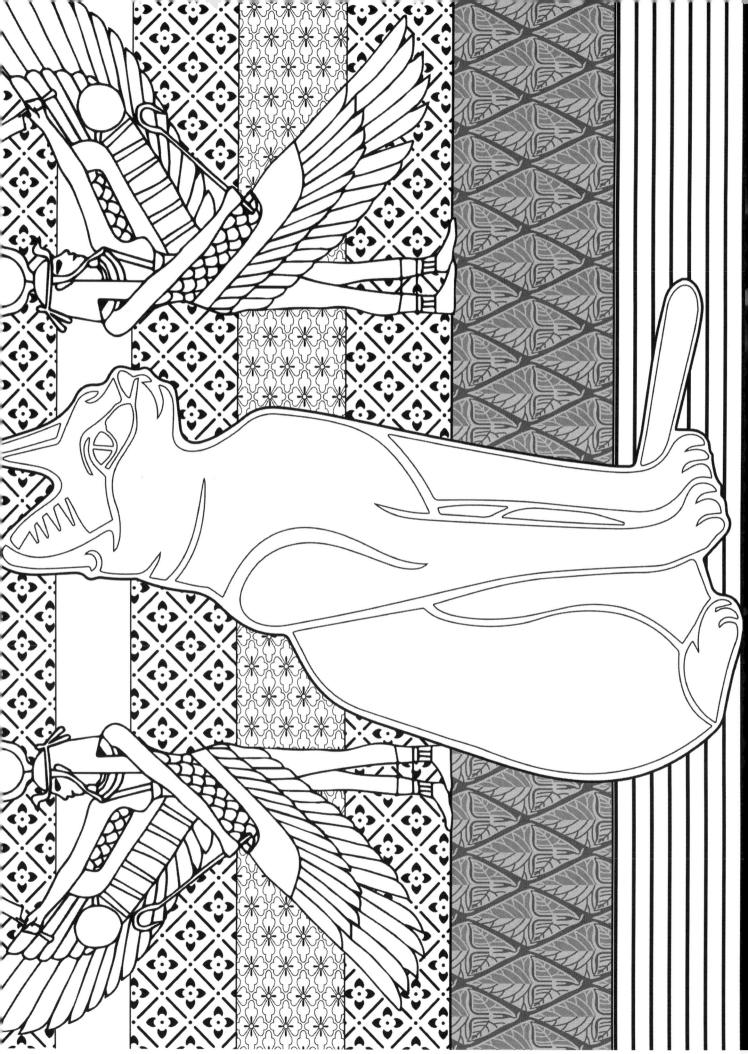

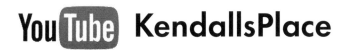

This page is left BLANK intentionally to avoid any bleed-through on the paper.

Thank you so much for purchasing my coloring book.
If you enjoyed this book please leave us a review on Amazon.

We want to see your drawings. Send us your colored version and tag us!

 @milehigherpod
@kendallraeonyt

@milehigherpodcast
@kendallraeonyt

"Perpetual **optimism** is a force multiplier. - **Colin Powell**

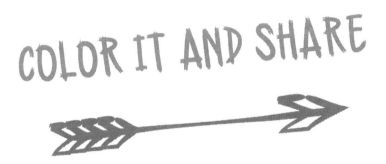

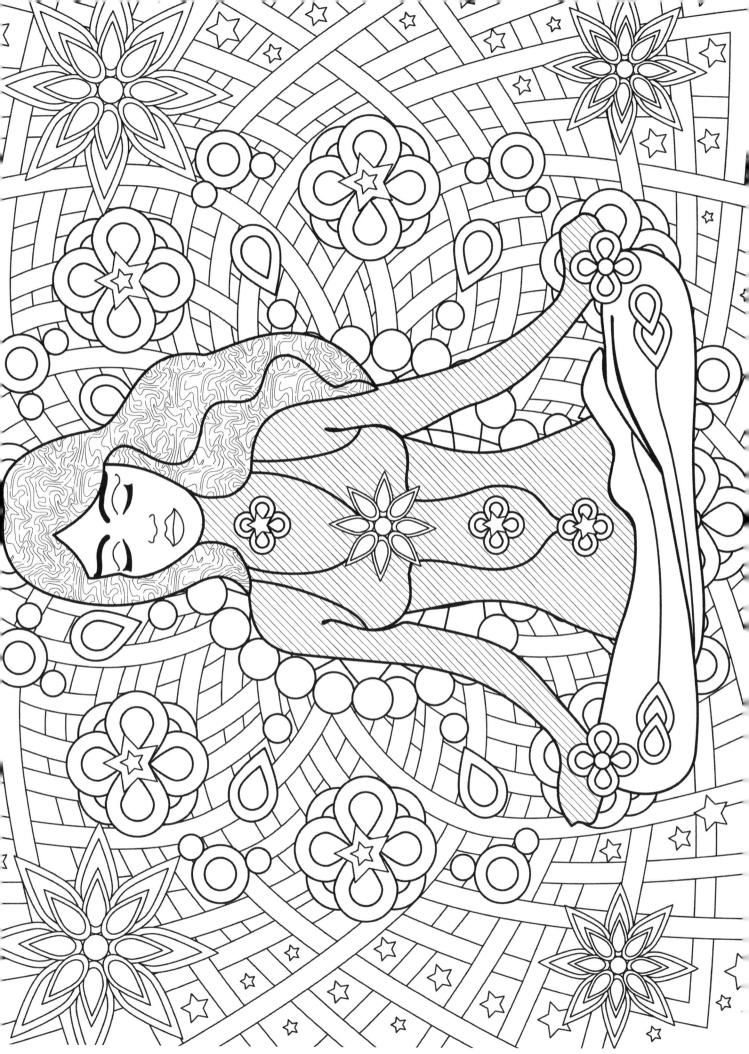

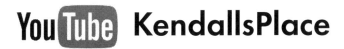

This page is left BLANK intentionally to avoid any bleed-through on the paper.

Thank you so much for purchasing my coloring book.
If you enjoyed this book please leave us a review on Amazon.

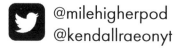
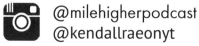

My dear friend clear your **mind** of can't. - **Samuel Johnson**

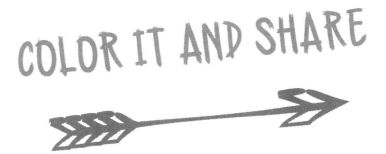

Want to get more free printable sheets? Get it here: **www.kendallr.com**

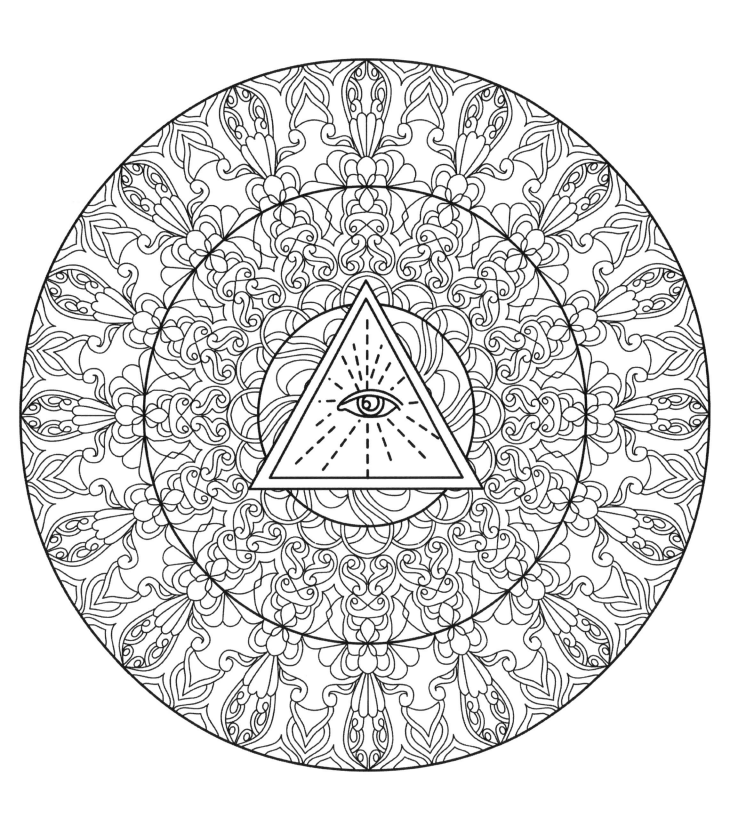

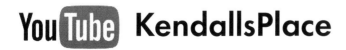

This page is left BLANK intentionally to avoid any bleed-through on the paper.

Thank you so much for purchasing my coloring book.
If you enjoyed this book please leave us a review on Amazon.

We want to see your drawings. Send us your colored version and tag us!

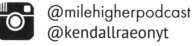

@milehigherpod
@kendallraeonyt

@milehigherpodcast
@kendallraeonyt

Be happy for this moment. This moment is your **life**. - **Omar Khayyam**

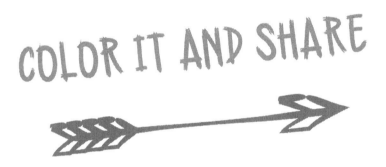

Want to get more free printable sheets? Get it here:
www.kendallr.com

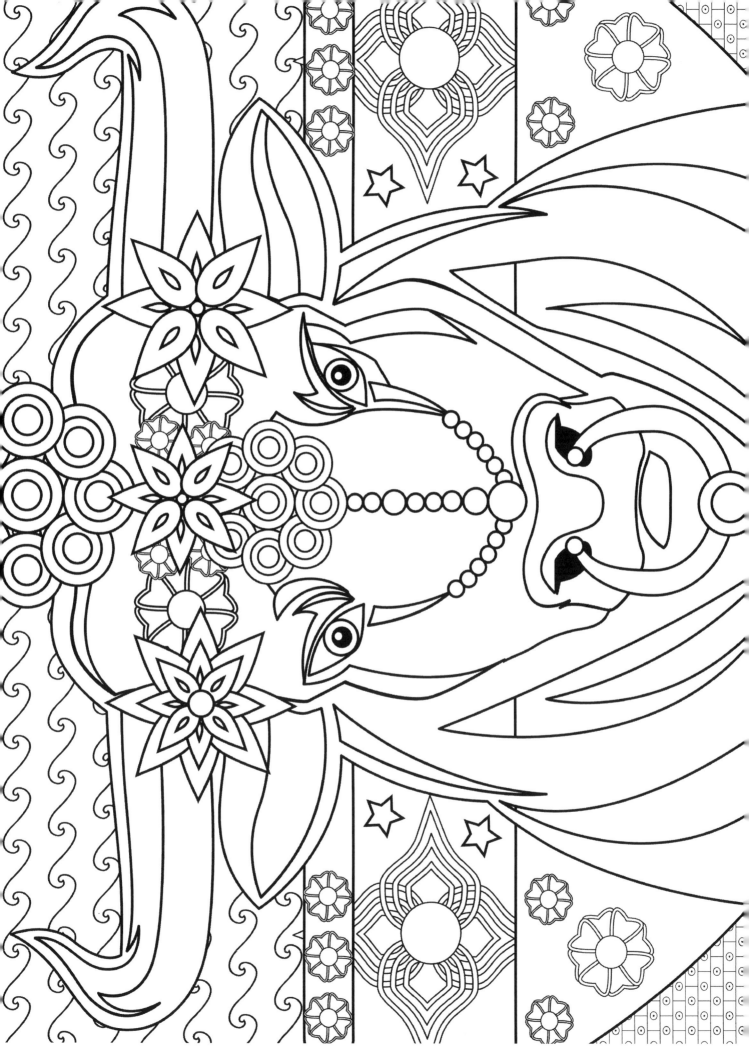

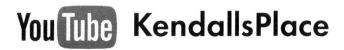

This page is left BLANK intentionally to avoid any bleed-through on the paper.

Thank you so much for purchasing my coloring book.
If you enjoyed this book please leave us a review on Amazon.

We want to see your drawings. Send us your colored version and tag us!

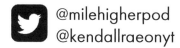 @milehigherpod
@kendallraeonyt

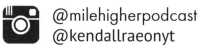 @milehigherpodcast
@kendallraeonyt

"

A **smile** is happiness you'll find right under your nose. - **Tom Wilson**

COLOR IT AND SHARE

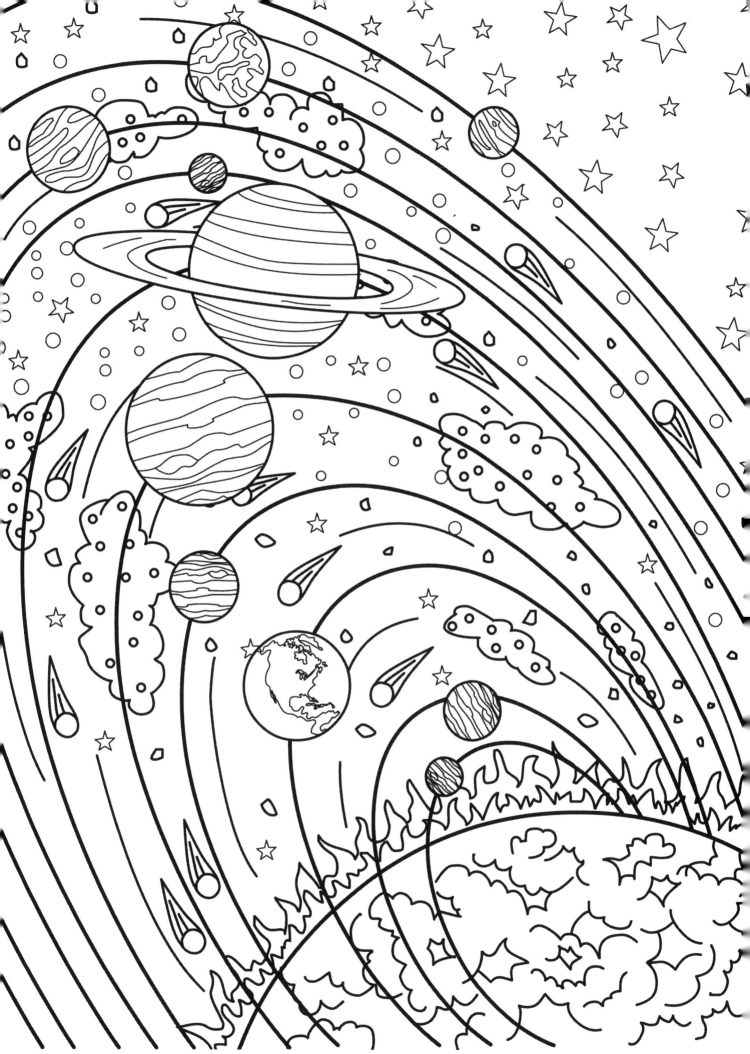

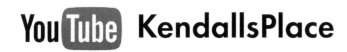

This page is left BLANK intentionally to avoid any bleed-through on the paper.

Thank you so much for purchasing my coloring book.
If you enjoyed this book please leave us a review on Amazon.

We want to see your drawings. Send us your colored version and tag us!

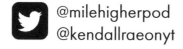 @milehigherpod
@kendallraeonyt

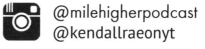 @milehigherpodcast
@kendallraeonyt

"

If you can not do great things, do small things in a **great way**. - **Napoleon Hill**

COLOR IT AND SHARE

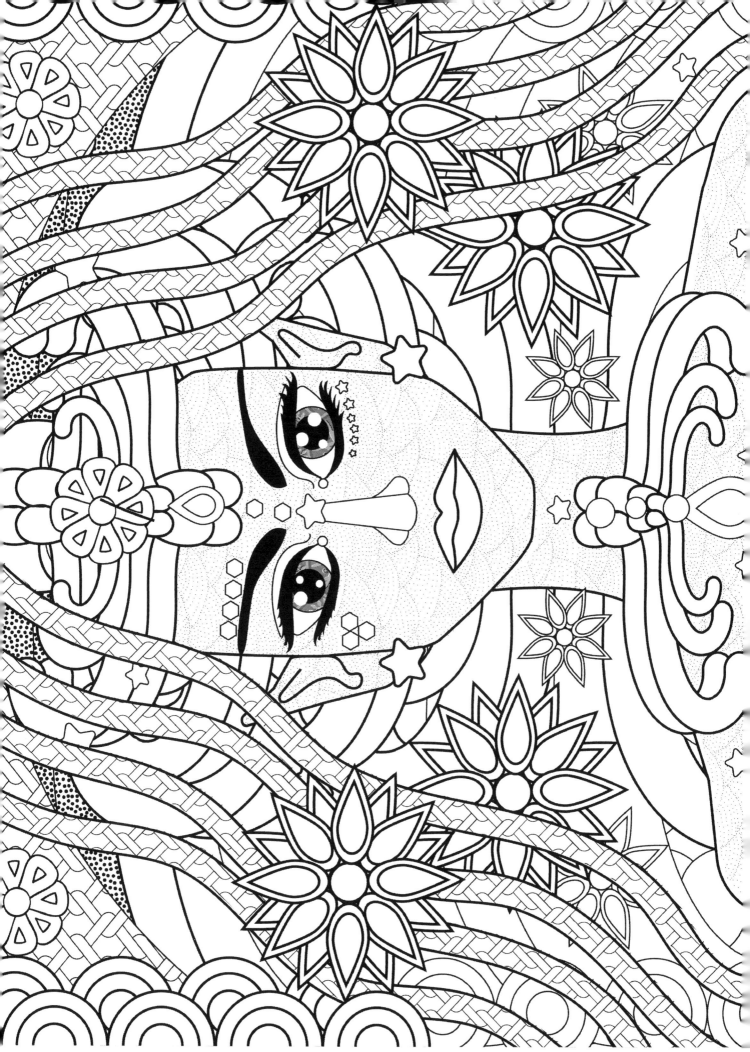

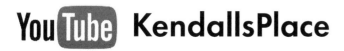

This page is left BLANK intentionally to avoid any bleed-through on the paper.

Thank you so much for purchasing my coloring book.
If you enjoyed this book please leave us a review on Amazon.

We want to see your drawings. Send us your colored version and tag us!

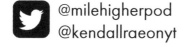 @milehigherpod
@kendallraeonyt

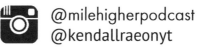 @milehigherpodcast
@kendallraeonyt

Someday is not a day of the week - **Denise Brennan-Nelson**

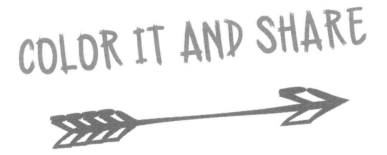

Want to get more free printable sheets? Get it here:
www.kendallr.com

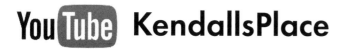

This page is left BLANK intentionally to avoid any bleed-through on the paper.

Thank you so much for purchasing my coloring book.
If you enjoyed this book please leave us a review on Amazon.

" Never **give up**, for that is just the place and time that the tide will turn. - **Harriet Beecher Stow**

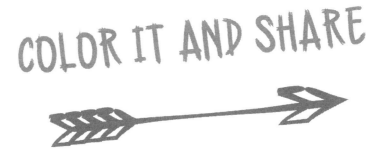

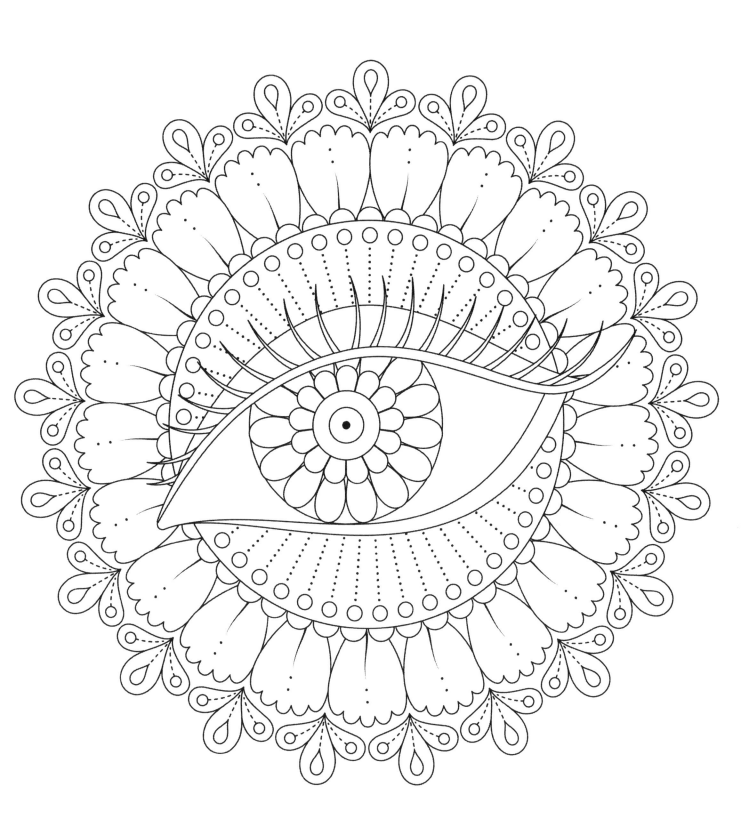

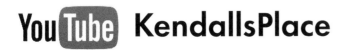

This page is left BLANK intentionally to avoid any bleed-through on the paper.

Thank you so much for purchasing my coloring book.
If you enjoyed this book please leave us a review on Amazon.

We want to see your drawings. Send us your colored version and tag us!

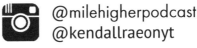

@milehigherpod   @milehigherpodcast
@kendallraeonyt   @kendallraeonyt

"

Adopt the pace of nature: her secret is patience - **Ralph Waldo Emerson**

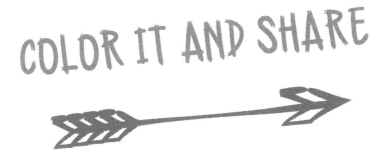

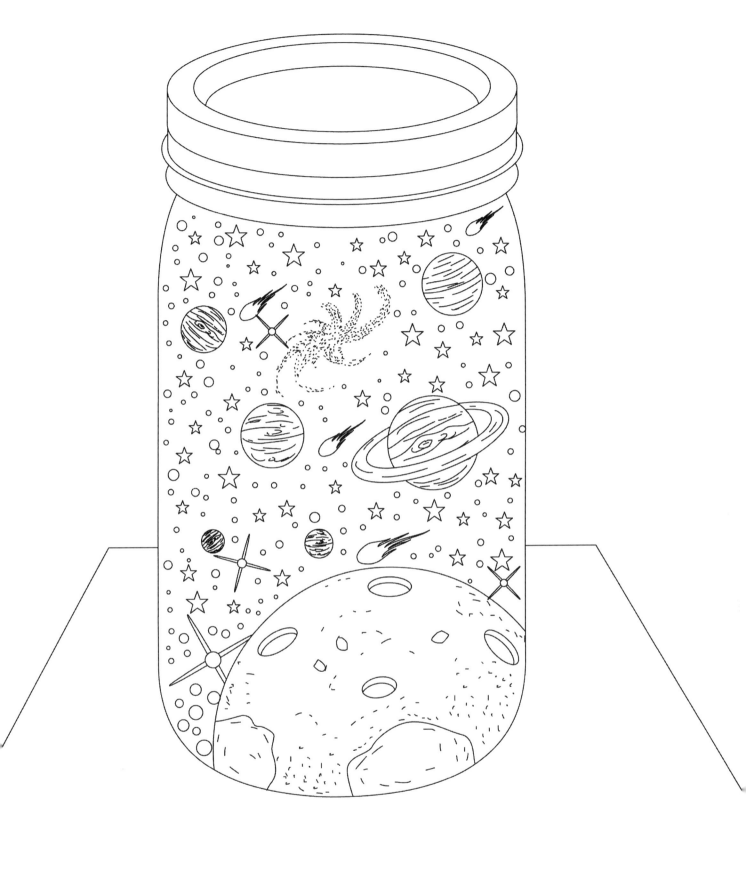

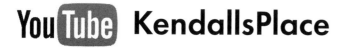

This page is left BLANK intentionally to avoid any bleed-through on the paper.

Thank you so much for purchasing my coloring book.
If you enjoyed this book please leave us a review on Amazon.

We want to see your drawings. Send us your colored version and tag us!

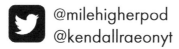 @milehigherpod
@kendallraeonyt

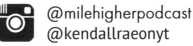 @milehigherpodcast
@kendallraeonyt

"

The best thing one can do when it's raining is to **let it rain**. - Henry Wadsworth Longfellow

COLOR IT AND SHARE

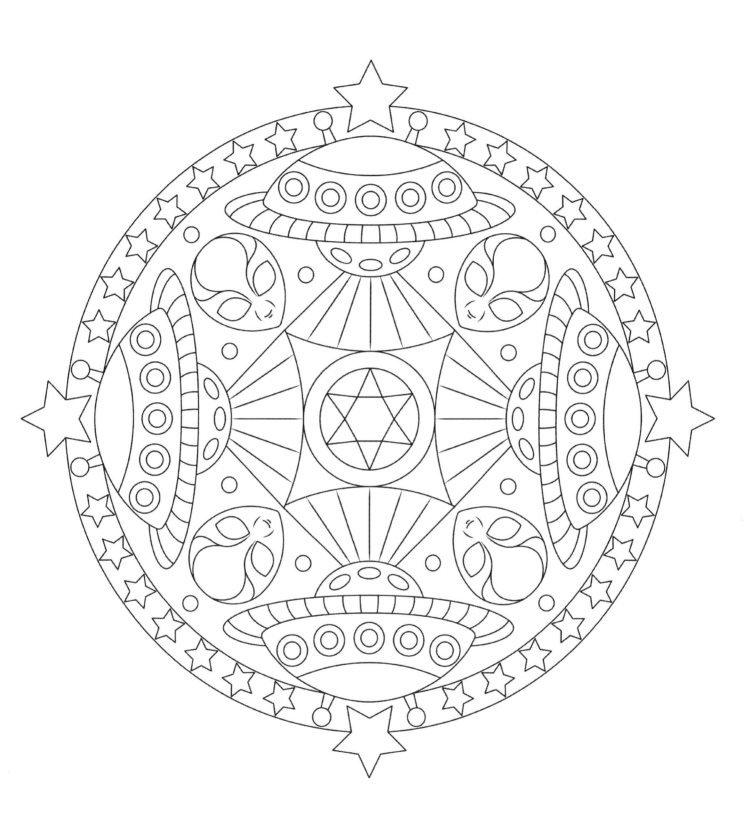

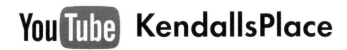

This page is left BLANK intentionally to avoid any bleed-through on the paper.

Thank you so much for purchasing my coloring book.
If you enjoyed this book please leave us a review on Amazon.

We want to see your drawings. Send us your colored version and tag us!

 @milehigherpod   @milehigherpodcast
@kendallraeonyt   @kendallraeonyt

" Deep in their roots, all flowers keep the light. -
Theodore Roethke

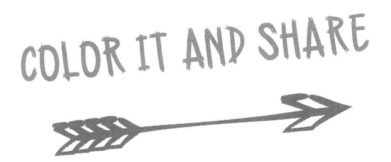

Want to get more free printable sheets? Get it here:
www.kendallr.com

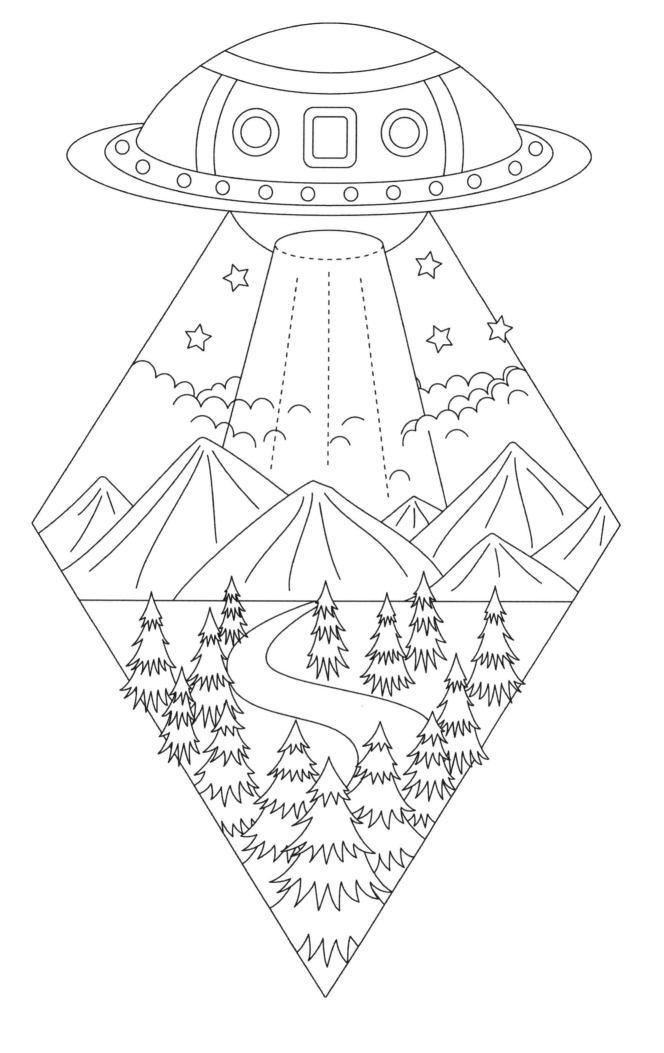